The Affordable Ketogenic Recipe Guide

Healthy and Tasty Ketogenic Recipes to Enjoy Your Diet and Boost Your Meals

Lauren Loose

© **Copyright 2021 - All rights reserved.**

The content contained within this book may not be reproduced, duplicated or transmitted without direct written permission from the author or the publisher.

Under no circumstances will any blame or legal responsibility be held against the publisher, or author, for any damages, reparation, or monetary loss due to the information contained within this book. Either directly or indirectly.

Legal Notice:

This book is copyright protected. This book is only for personal use. You cannot amend, distribute, sell, use, quote or paraphrase any part, or the content within this book, without the consent of the author or publisher.

Disclaimer Notice:

Please note the information contained within this document is for educational and entertainment purposes only. All effort has been executed to present accurate, up to date, and reliable, complete information. No warranties of any kind are declared or implied. Readers acknowledge that the author is not engaging in the rendering of legal, financial, medical or professional advice. The content within this book has been derived from various sources. Please consult a licensed professional before attempting any techniques outlined in this book.

By reading this document, the reader agrees that under no circumstances is the author responsible for any losses, direct or indirect, which are incurred as a result of the use of information contained within this document, including, but not limited to, — errors, omissions, or inaccuracies.

Contents

Ketogenic Sloppy Joes 7

Low Carb Crack Slaw Egg Roll in a Bowl Recipe 9

Low Carb Beef Stir Fry 11

One Pan Pesto Chicken and Veggies 13

Crispy Peanut Tofu and Cauliflower Rice Stir-Fry 15

Simple Ketogenic Fried Chicken 18

Ketogenic Butter Chicken 21

Ketogenic Shrimp Scampi Recipe 23

Ketogenic Lasagna 25

Creamy Tuscan Garlic Chicken 28

Almond Butter Muffins 30

Classic Western Omelet 32

Sheet Pan Eggs with Ham   and Pepper Jack 34

Tomato Mozzarella   Egg Muffins 36

Crispy Chai Waffles 38

Broccoli, Kale, Egg Scramble 40

Three Cheese Egg Muffins 42

Bacon, Mushroom,   and Swiss Omelet 44

Coco-Cashew   Macadamia Muffins 46

Maple Cranberry Muffins 48

Chocolate Protein Pancakes 50

Beef and Eggplant Kebab 52

Skin Salmon with Pesto Cauliflower Rice 54

Chicken Enchilada Casserole 56

Ketogenic Cottage Pie 58

Pan Fried Spinach Stuffed Chicken 61

Ketogenic Chicken Tenders	63
Low-Carb Salmon Tray Bake	65
Zesty Low-Carb Chicken Tacos	67
Ketogenic Chicken Doner Kebabs	69
Low-Carb Instant Pot Frittata	71
Balsamic Chicken Thighs	73
Chicken Marsala	75
Chicken Fajitas	77
Spring Beef Bourguignon	79
Mexican Shredded Beef	81
Pork Tenderloin	83
Creamy Lemon Chicken	85
Asian Porkchops	87
Sausage and Peppers	88
Low-Carb Beef Short Ribs	90
Zucchini Lasagna with Meat Sauce	92
Chinese Pulled Pork – Char Siu	95
Garlic Butter Chicken with Cream Cheese Sauce	97
Spinach Artichoke Chicken	99
Bacon Wrapped Pork Loin	100
Chicken Cordon Bleu with Cauliflower	101
Sesame-Crusted Tuna with Green Beans	103
Rosemary Roasted Pork with Cauliflower	105
Grilled Salmon and Zucchini with Mango Sauce	107

Ketogenic Sloppy Joes

Total time: 45 minutes

Ingredients :

1 ¼ cup almond flour (for the bread)

5 tbsp. ground psyllium husk powder (for the bread)

1 tsp. sea salt (for the bread)

2 tsp. baking powder (for the bread)

2 tsp. cider vinegar (for the bread)

1 ¼ cups boiling water (for the bread)

3 egg whites (for the bread)

2 tbsp. olive oil (for the meat sauce)

1 ½ lbs. ground beef (for the meat sauce)

1 yellow onion (for the meat sauce)

4 garlic cloves (for the meat sauce)

14 oz. crushed tomatoes (for the meat sauce)

1 tbsp. chili powder (for the meat sauce)

1 tbsp. Dijon powder (for the meat sauce)

1 tbsp. red wine vinegar (for the meat sauce)

4 tbsp. tomato paste (for the meat sauce)

2 tsp. salt (for the meat sauce)

¼ tsp ground black pepper (for the meat sauce)

½ cup mayonnaise as toppings

6 oz. shredded cheese as toppings

Directions:

We are going to start by cooking the bread. First, preheat the 350 degrees Fahrenheit and then mix all the dry ingredients in a bowl.

Add some vinegar, egg whites, and boiling water in the bowl. Whisk thoroughly for 30 seconds or use a hand mixer to speed up the process. You would want a consistency that is a lot like playday

Form the dough into 5 or 8 pieces of bread. Layer then on the lowest oven rack and cook for 55 to 60 minutes.

In the meantime, you will be cooking the meat sauce. Grab a pan and cook the onion and garlic until you get that fragrant smell.

Add the ground beef and cook the meat thoroughly. Once done, add the other ingredients and cook

Allow it to simmer for 10 minutes in low heat. Add other seasonings to taste.

Low Carb Crack Slaw Egg Roll in a Bowl Recipe

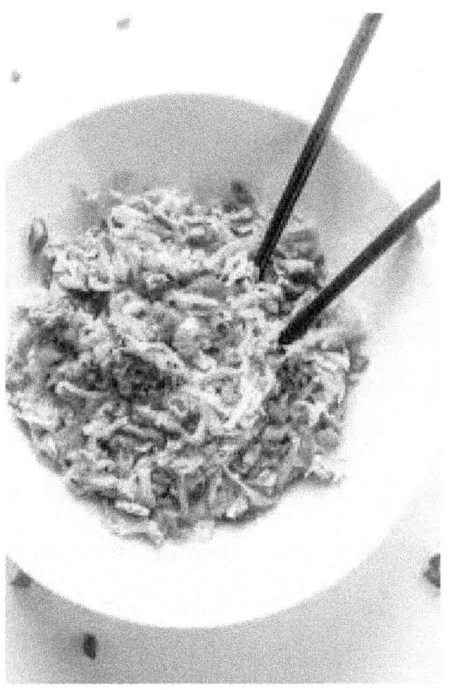

Total time: 20 minutes

Ingredients :

1 lb. ground beef

4 cups shredded coleslaw mix

1 tbsp. avocado oil

1 tsp. sea salt

¼ tsp. black pepper

4 cloves garlic, minced

3 tbsp. fresh ginger, grated

¼ cup coconut amines

2 tsp. toasted sesame oil

¼ cup green onions

Directions:

Start by heating the avocado oil in a large pan using a medium-high heat. Put in the garlic and cook for a little bit until you get that fragrant smell.

Add the ground beef and cook until it gets brownish. This should take about 10 minutes to finish. Season with salt and black pepper.

Once cooked, you can lower the heat and add the coleslaw mix and the coconut amines. Stir to cook for 5 minutes or until the coleslaw gets tender.

Remove and put in the green onions and the toasted sesame oil.

Low Carb Beef Stir Fry

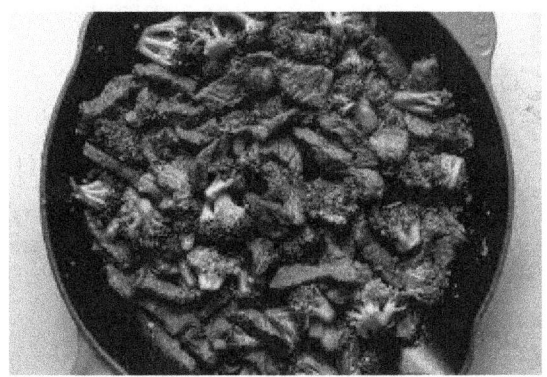

Total time: 25 minutes

Ingredients :

½ cup zucchini, spiral them into noodles about 6-inches each

¼ cup organic broccoli florets

1 bunch baby book choy, stem chopped

2 tbsp. avocado oil

2 tsp. coconut amines

1 small know of ginger, peeled, and cut

8 oz. skirt steak, thinly sliced into strips

Directions:

Heat the pan and add 1 tablespoon of oil. Sear the steak on it on high heat. This should only take around 2 minutes per side.

Reduce the heat to medium and put in the broccoli, ginger, ghee, and coconut amines. Cook for a minute, stirring as often as possible.

Add in the book choy and cook for another minute

Finally, put the zucchini into the mix and cook. Note that zucchini noodles cook quickly so you would want to pay close attention to this.

One Pan Pesto Chicken and Veggies

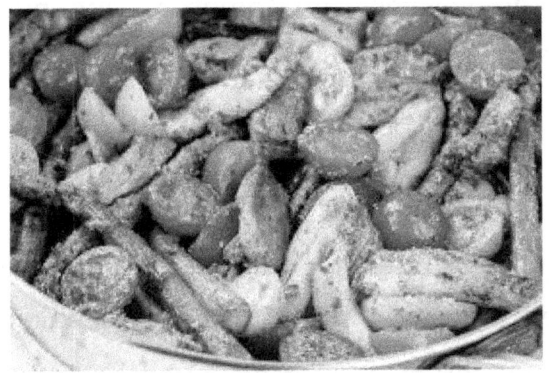

Total time: 35 minutes

Ingredients :

2 tbsp. olive oil

1 cup cherry diced tomatoes

¼ cup basil pesto

1/3 cup sun-dried tomatoes, chopped and drained

1-pound chicken thigh, bones and skinless, sliced into strips

1-pound asparagus, cut in half with the ends trimmed

Directions:

Start by heating up a large skillet. Put two tablespoons of olive oil and sliced chicken on medium heat. Season with salt and add ½ cup of the sun-dried tomatoes.

Cook for a few minutes until the chicken is cooked thoroughly. Spoon out the chicken and tomatoes and put them in a separate container.

Do not wash the skillet just yet. You will be using the oil there later.

Next, put the asparagus in the skillet and pour in the pesto. Turn the heat on medium and add the remaining sun-dried tomatoes. Cook the asparagus for 5 to 10 minutes. Put it on a separate plate when done.

Put the chicken back in the skillet and pour in pesto. Stir under medium heat for 2 minutes. You only need to reheat the chicken during this so when done, you can serve it together with the asparagus.

Crispy Peanut Tofu and Cauliflower Rice Stir-Fry

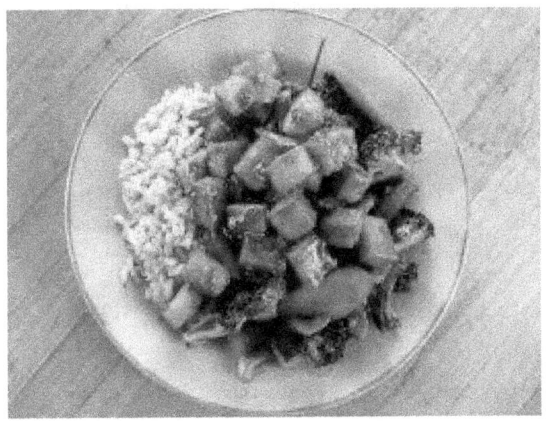

Total time: 1 hour 35 minutes

Ingredients :

12 oz. tofu, extra-firm

1 tbsp. toasted sesame oil

2 cloves minced garlic

1 small cauliflower head

1 ½ tbsp. toasted sesame oil (sauce)

½ tsp. chili garlic sauce (sauce)

2 ½ tbsp. peanut butter (sauce)

¼ cup low sodium soy sauce (sauce)

½ cup light brown sugar (sauce)

Directions:

Start by draining the tofu for 90 minutes before getting the meal ready. You can dry the tofu quickly by rolling it on an absorbent towel and putting something heavy on top. This will create a gentle pressure on the tofu to drain out the water.

Preheat the oven to 400 degrees Fahrenheit. While the oven heats up, cube the tofu, and prepare your baking sheet.

Bake for 25 minutes and allow it to cool.

Combine the sauce ingredients and whisk it thoroughly until you get that well-blended texture. You can add more ingredients, depending on your personal preferences with taste.

Put the tofu in the sauce and stir it quickly to coat the tofu thoroughly. Leave it there for 15 minutes or more for a thorough marinate.

While the tofu marinates, shred the cauliflower into rice- size bits. You can also try buying cauliflower rice from the store to save yourself this step. If you are doing this manually, use a fine grater or a food processor.

Grab a skillet and put it on medium heat. Start cooking the veggies on a bit of sesame oil and just a little bit of soy sauce. Set it aside.

Grab the tofu and put it on the pan. Stir the tofu frequently until it gets that nice golden-brown color. Do not worry if some of the tofu sticks to the pan – it will do that sometimes. Set aside.

Steam your cauliflower rice for 5 to 8 minutes. Add some sauce and stir thoroughly.

Now it is time to add up the ingredients together. Put the cauliflower rice with the veggies and tofu. Serve and enjoy. You can reheat this if there are leftovers but try not to leave it in the fridge for long.

Simple Ketogenic Fried Chicken

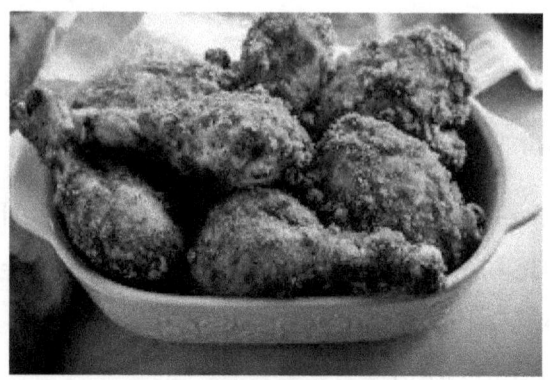

Total time: 45 minutes

Ingredients :

4 boneless and skinless chicken thighs

Frying oil

2 large eggs

2 tbsp. heavy whipping cream

2/3 cup grated parmesan cheese (breading)

2/3 cup blanched almond flour (breading)

1 tsp. salt (breading)

½ tsp. black pepper (breading)

½ tsp. cayenne (breading)

½ tsp. paprika (breading)

Directions:

Grab a bowl and put together the eggs and heavy cream. Beat them together until perfectly mixed.

Grab another bowl, this time combining all the breading ingredients and mix well. Set it aside for now.

Cut the chicken thigh into 3 even pieces. Make sure they are not wet by patting the moist area with a paper towel. This will help prevent the oil splashes when you start frying them.

So now you have the chicken and 2 bowls. One bowl contains the egg wash and the other contains the breading. Dip the chicken in the bread first before dipping it in the egg wash and then finally, dipping it in the breading again. Make sure it is completely covered.

Put 2 inches worth of oil in a pot and heat it up until it reaches around 350 degrees Fahrenheit or when it starts to become steamy. When this happens, try to gradually lower the heat so you can maintain that temperature. This is important since a perfectly heated oil will help create crunchy chicken.

Put the coated chicken in your hot oil. Do this gently with a pair of tongs, making sure there are no splashes of any kind. Frying time should take around 5 minutes or until the coating becomes deep brown in color.

Prepare some paper towels and put the cooked chicken on it. This will help remove any excess oil.

Try not to overcrowd the pan so all of them will cook beautifully. Serve while still crispy for best results.

Ketogenic Butter Chicken

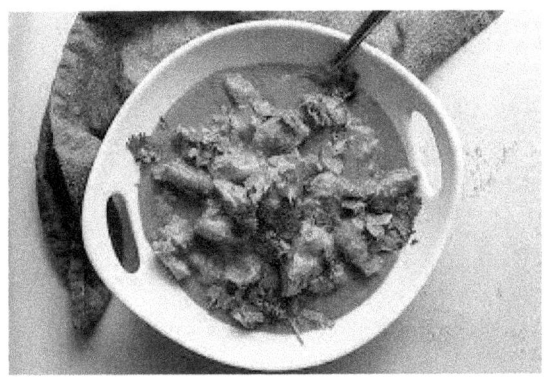

Total time: 35 minutes

Ingredients :

1.5 lb. chicken breast

1 tbsp. coconut oil

2 tbsp. garam masala

3 tsp. grated fresh ginger

3 tsp. minced garlic

4 oz. plain yogurt

2 tbsp. butter (for sauce)

1 tbsp. ground coriander (for sauce)

½ cup heavy cream (for sauce)

½ tbsp. garam masala (for sauce)

2 tsp. fresh ginger, grated (for sauce)

2 tsp. minced garlic (for sauce)

2 tsp. cumin (for sauce)

1 tsp. chili powder (for sauce)

1 onion (for sauce)

14.5 oz. crushed tomatoes (for sauce)

Salt to taste (for sauce)

Directions:

Start by cutting the chicken into pieces measuring around 2 inches each. Place it in a large bowl and add 2 tablespoons of garam masala, 1 teaspoon of minced garlic, and 1 teaspoon of grated ginger. Stir slowly and add the yogurt. Make sure that mix is evenly distributed before putting a lid on the container and chilling it in the fridge for 30 minutes.

For the sauce, grab a blender and put in the ginger, garlic, onion, tomatoes, and spices. Blend until smooth.

Leave the blended sauce aside and grab a skillet. Using medium heat, remove the chicken from the fridge and cook, allowing it to brown on both sides.

Once cooked, pour in the sauce, and allow it to simmer for 5 more minutes

Finally, put in the cream and ghee, still using medium heat. Add some salt for taste and serve!

Ketogenic Shrimp Scampi Recipe

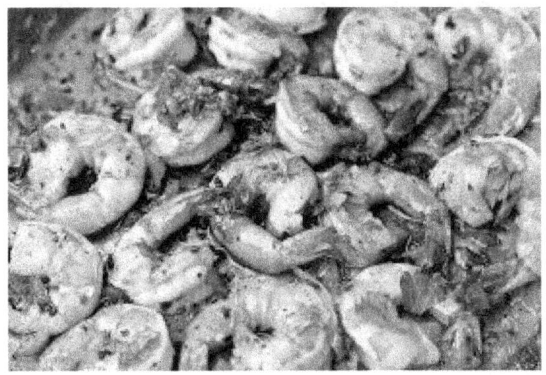

Total time: 35 minutes

Ingredients :

2 summer squash

1-pound shrimp, deveined

2 tbsp. butter unsalted

2 tbsp. lemon juice

2 tbsp. chopped parsley

¼ cup chicken broth

1/8 tsp. red chili flakes

1 clove minced garlic

Salt and pepper to taste

Directions:

Start by cutting the summer squash into noodle-like shapes. You can use a spiralizer to get this done or perhaps use a fork to scrap the surface.

Spread the noodles on top of paper towards and sprinkle them with salt. Set aside for 30 minutes.

Blot the excess water with a paper towel.

In a frying pan, melt butter over medium heat and fry the garlic until you get that fragrant smell. Add some chicken broth, red chili flakes, and lemon juice.

Once it boils, add the shrimp, and allow it to cook. Reduce the heat once the shrimp turns pink.

Add more salt and pepper to taste before adding the summer squash noodles and parsley to the mix. Make sure all the ingredients are well-coated by the sauce. Serve.

Ketogenic Lasagna

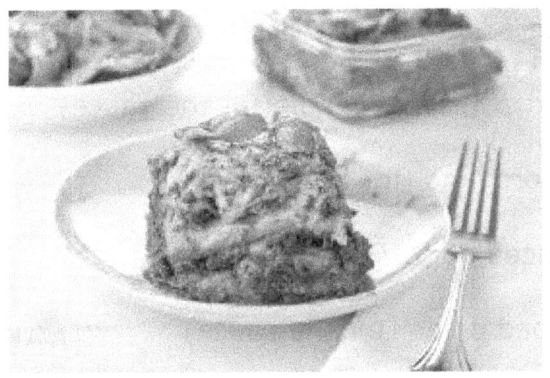

Total time: 1 hour 35 minutes

Ingredients :

8 oz. block of cream cheese

3 large eggs

Kosher salt

Ground black pepper

2 cups of shredded mozzarella

½ cup of freshly grated parmesan

Pinch crushed red pepper flakes

Chopped parsley for garnish

¾ cup marinara (for the sauce)

1 tbsp. tomato paste (for the sauce)

1 lb. ground beef (for the sauce)

½ cup of freshly grated parmesan (for the sauce)

1.5 cup of shredded mozzarella (for the sauce)

1 tbsp. of extra virgin olive oil (for the sauce)

1 tsp. dried oregano (for the sauce)

3 cloves minced garlic (for the sauce)

½ cup chopped onion (for the sauce)

16 oz. ricotta (for the sauce)

Directions:

Start by preheating the oven to 350 degrees and preparing the baking tray by lining it with parchment and cooking spray.

Grab a microwave-safe bowl and throw in the cream cheese, mozzarella, and parmesan, melting them together for a few seconds in the microwave. Mix them in thoroughly before adding the eggs and blending the whole thing together. Add a pinch of salt and pepper for seasoning.

Spread the mixture on a baking sheet and bake for 15 to 20 minutes.

While baking, grab a skillet and using medium heat, coat the surface with oil. Put in the onion and allow them to cook for 5 minutes before adding the garlic. Once you get that fragrant smell, wait 60 more seconds before adding the tomato paste onto the mixture. Make sure to stir all the items around until the onion and garlic are well-coated.

Add the ground beef in the skillet and cook the mixture, breaking up the meat until it is no longer pinks in appearance. Add salt and pepper to taste. Cook it for a few more minutes before setting it aside and allowing it to cool. There should be a bit of fluid remaining in the skillet – try to drain that out of the meat before proceeding with the next step.

Turn on the stove again, keeping the medium heat constant. Add some marinara sauce and season with pepper, red pepper flakes, and ground pepper. Stir around to evenly distribute the flavor.

By this time, your noodles should be ready from the oven. Take them out and start cutting them in half widthwise and then cut them again into 3 pieces.

Start layering! Use an 8-inch baking pan for this, placing 2 noodles at the bottom of the dish first and layer as you wish. Alternate the parmesan and mozzarella shreds depending on your personal preferences.

Bake until the cheese melts and the sauce bubbles out. Should take about 30 minutes.

Garnish and serve.

Creamy Tuscan Garlic Chicken

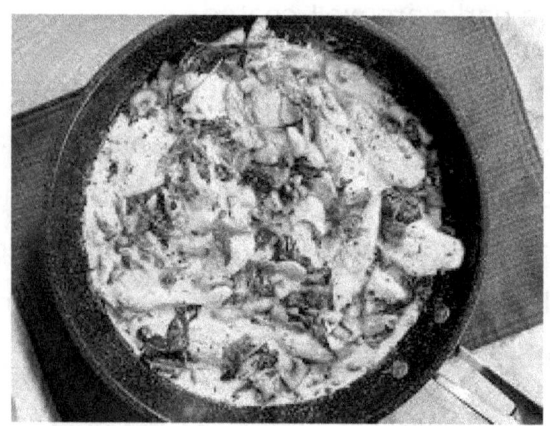

Total time: 30 minutes

Ingredients :

1.5 pounds boneless and skinless chicken breast, thinly sliced

½ cup chicken broth

½ cup parmesan cheese

½ cup sun dried tomatoes

1 cup heavy cream

1 cup chopped spinach

2 tbsp. olive oil

1 tsp. garlic powder

1 tsp. Italian seasoning

Directions:

Grab a large skillet and cook the chicken using olive oil using medium heat. Do this for 5 minutes for each side or until they are thoroughly cooked. Set it aside in a plate.

Using the same skillet, combine the heavy cream, garlic powder, Italian seasoning, parmesan cheese, and chicken broth. Expose it to medium heat and just whisk away until the mixture thickens.

Add the sundried tomatoes and spinach and let it simmer until the spinach wilts.

Add the chicken back and serve.

Almond Butter Muffins

Preparation Time: 10 minutes

Cooking Time: 25 minutes

Servings: 6

Ingredients:

1cups almond flour

1/2 cup powdered erythritol

1 teaspoon baking powder

¼ teaspoon salt

¾ cup almond butter, warmed.

¾ cup unsweetened almond milk

2 large eggs

Directions:

Preheat the oven to 350 ° F, and line a paper liner muffin pan.

In a mixing bowl, whisk the almond flour and the erythritol, baking powder, and salt.

Whisk the almond milk, almond butter, and the eggs together in a separate bowl.

Drop the wet ingredients into the dry until just mixed.

Spoon the batter into the prepared pan and bake for 22 to 25 minutes until clean comes out the knife inserted in the middle.

Cook the muffins in the pan for 5 minutes. Then, switch onto a cooling rack with wire.

Nutrition:

Calories: 135 kcal

Fat: 11g

Protein: 6g

Carbohydrates: 4g

Fiber: 2g

Net carbs: 2g

Classic Western Omelet

Preparation Time: 5 minutes

Cooking Time: 10 minutes

Servings: 1

Ingredients:

2 teaspoons coconut oil

3 large eggs, whisked.

1 tablespoon heavy cream

Salt and pepper

¼ cup diced green pepper.

¼ cup diced yellow onion.

¼ cup diced ham.

Directions:

In a small bowl, whisk the eggs, heavy cream, salt, and pepper.

Heat up 1 teaspoon of coconut oil over medium heat in a small skillet.

Add the peppers and onions, then sauté the ham for 3 to 4 minutes.

Spoon the mixture in a cup and heat the skillet with the remaining oil.

Pour in the whisked eggs and cook until the egg's bottom begins to set.

Tilt the pan and cook until almost set to spread the egg.

Spoon the ham and veggie mixture over half of the omelet and turn over.

Let cook the omelet until the eggs are set and then serve hot.

Nutrition:

Calories: 415 kcal

Fat: 32.5g

Protein: 25g

Carbs: 6.5g

Sugar: 1.5g

Net carbohydrates: 5g

Sheet Pan Eggs with Ham and Pepper Jack

Preparation Time: 5 minutes

Cooking Time: 15 minutes

Servings: 6

Ingredients:

12 large eggs, whisked.

Salt and pepper

2 cups diced ham.

1 cup shredded pepper jack cheese

Directions:

Preheat the oven to 350°F and grease a rimmed baking sheet with cooking spray.

Whisk the eggs in a mixing bowl then add salt and pepper until frothy.

Stir in the ham and cheese and mix until well combined.

Pour the mixture in baking sheets and spread into an even layer.

Bake for 12 to 15 minutes until the egg is set.

Let cool slightly then cut it into squares to serve.

Nutrition:

Calories: 235 kcal

Fat: 15g

Protein: 21g

Carbs: 2.5g

Fiber: 0.5g

Net carbs: 2g

Tomato Mozzarella Egg Muffins

Preparation Time: 5 minutes

Cooking Time: 25 minutes

Servings: 12

Ingredients:

1 tablespoon butter

1 medium tomato finely diced.

½ cup diced yellow onion.

12 large eggs, whisked.

½ cup canned coconut milk

¼ cup sliced green onion.

Salt and pepper

1 cup shredded mozzarella cheese

Directions:

Preheat the oven to 350 ° F and grease the cooking spray into a muffin pan.

Melt the butter over moderate heat in a medium skillet.

Add the tomato and onions, then cook until softened for 3 to 4 minutes.

Divide the mix between cups of muffins.

Whisk the bacon, coconut milk, green onions, salt, and pepper together and then spoon into the muffin cups.

Sprinkle with cheese until the egg is set, then bake for 15 to 25 minutes.

Nutrition:

Calories: 135 kcal

Fat: 10.5g

Protein: 9g

Carbs: 2g

Fiber: 0.5g

Net carbs: 1.5g

Crispy Chai Waffles

Preparation Time: 10 minutes

Cooking Time: 20 minutes

Servings: 4

Ingredients:

4 large eggs separated into whites and yolks.

3 tablespoons coconut flour

3 tablespoons powdered erythritol

1 ¼ teaspoon baking powder

1 teaspoon vanilla extract

½ teaspoon ground cinnamon

¼ teaspoon ground ginger

Pinch ground cloves

Pinch ground cardamom

3 tablespoons coconut oil, melted.

3 tablespoons unsweetened almond milk

Directions:

Divide the eggs into two separate mixing bowls.

Whip the whites of the eggs until stiff peaks develop and then set aside.

Whisk the egg yolks into the other bowl with the coconut flour, erythritol, baking powder, cocoa, cinnamon, cardamom, and cloves.

Pour the melted coconut oil and the almond milk into the second bowl and whisk.

Fold softly in the whites of the egg until you have just combined.

Preheat waffle iron with cooking spray and grease.

Spoon into the iron for about 1/2 cup of batter

Cook the waffle according to directions from the maker.

Move the waffle to a plate and repeat with the batter left over.

Nutrition:

Calories: 215 kcal

Fat: 17g

Protein: 8g

Carbohydrates: 8g

Fiber: 4g

Net carbs: 4g

Broccoli, Kale, Egg Scramble

Preparation Time: 5 minutes

Cooking Time: 10 minutes

Servings: 1

Ingredients:

2 large eggs, whisked.

1 tablespoon heavy cream

Salt and pepper

1 teaspoon coconut oil

1 cup fresh chopped kale

¼ cup frozen broccoli florets, thawed.

2 tablespoons grated parmesan cheese

Directions:

In a mug, whisk the eggs along with the heavy cream, salt, and pepper.

Heat 1 teaspoon coconut oil over medium heat in a medium-size skillet.

Stir in the kale and broccoli, then cook about 1 to 2 minutes until the kale is wilted.

Pour in the eggs and cook until just set, stirring occasionally.

Stir in the cheese with parmesan and serve hot.

Nutrition:

Calories: 315 kcal

Fat: 25g

Protein: 19.5g

Carbs: 10g

Fiber: 1.5g

net carbs: 8.5g

Three Cheese Egg Muffins

Preparation Time: 5 minutes

Cooking Time: 20 minutes

Servings: 8

Ingredients:

1 tablespoon butter

½ cup diced yellow onion.

12 large eggs, whisked.

½ cup canned coconut milk

¼ cup sliced green onion.

Salt and pepper

½ cup shredded cheddar cheese

½ cup shredded Swiss cheese.

¼ cup grated parmesan cheese

Directions:

Preheat the oven to 350 ° F and grease the cooking spray into a muffin pan.

Melt the butter over moderate heat in a medium skillet.

Add the onions then cook until softened for 3 to 4 minutes.

Divide the mix between cups of muffins.

Whisk the bacon, coconut milk, green onions, salt, and pepper together and then spoon into the muffin cups.

In a cup, mix the three kinds of cheese, and scatter over the egg muffins.

Bake till the egg is set, for 20 to 25 minutes.

Nutrition:

Calories: 150 kcal

Fat: 11.5g

Protein: 10g

Carbs: 2g

Fiber: 0.5g

net carbs: 1.5g

Bacon, Mushroom, and Swiss Omelet

Preparation Time: 5 minutes

Cooking Time: 10 minutes

Servings: 1

Ingredients:

3 large eggs, whisked.

1 tablespoon heavy cream

Salt and pepper

2 slices uncooked bacon, chopped.

¼ cup diced mushrooms.

¼ cup shredded Swiss cheese.

Directions:

Whisk the eggs together in a small bowl with heavy cream, salt, and pepper.

Cook the bacon over medium to high heat in a small skillet.

Spoon it in a mug when the bacon is crisp.

Steam the skillet over medium heat, then add the chestnuts.

Cook the mushrooms until they smoke, then spoon the bacon into the dish.

Heat the skillet with the remaining oil.

Pour in the whisked eggs and cook until the egg's bottom begins to set.

To scatter the egg, tilt the saucepan and cook until almost set.

Spoon the mixture of bacon and mushroom over half of the omelet, then sprinkle with the cheese and fold over.

Let the omelet cook until the eggs have been set and serve hot.

Nutrition:

Calories: 475 kcal

Fat: 36g

Protein: 34g

Carbohydrates: 4g

Fiber: 0.5g

Net carbs: 3.5g

Coco-Cashew Macadamia Muffins

Preparation Time: 10 minutes

Cooking Time: 25 minutes

Servings: 12

Ingredients:

1 ¾ cups almond flour

1 cup powdered erythritol

¼ cup unsweetened cocoa powder

2 teaspoons baking powder.

¼ teaspoon salt

¾ cup cashew butter, melted.

¾ cup unsweetened almond milk

4 large eggs

¼ cup chopped macadamia nuts.

Directions:

Preheat the oven to 350 ° F and use paper liners to line a muffin pan.

In a mixing bowl, whisk the almond flour along with the erythritol, cocoa powder, baking powder, and salt.

Whisk the almond milk, the cashew butter, and the eggs together in a separate bowl.

Move the wet ingredients to the dry when mixed, then insert into the nuts.

Spoon the batter into the prepared pan and bake for 22 to 25 minutes until clean comes out the knife inserted in the middle.

Cook the muffins in the pan for 5 minutes, and then switch onto a cooling rack with wire.

Nutrition:

Calories: 230g

Fat: 20g

Protein: 9g

Carbohydrates: 9g

Fiber: 2.5g

Net carbs: 6.5g

Maple Cranberry Muffins

Preparation Time: 10 minutes

Cooking Time: 20 minutes

Servings: 12

Ingredients:

¾ cups almond flour

¼ cup ground flaxseed

¼ cup powdered erythritol

1 teaspoon baking powder

⅛ teaspoon salt

⅓ cup canned coconut milk

¼ cup coconut oil, melted.

3 large eggs

½ cup fresh cranberries

1 teaspoon maple extract

Directions:

Preheat the oven to 350 ° F, and line a paper liner muffin pan.

In a mixing bowl, whisk the almond flour along with the ground flaxseed, erythritol, baking powder, and salt.

Whisk coconut milk, coconut oil, eggs, and maple extract together in a separate bowl.

Move the wet ingredients to the dry until just full, then fold into the cranberries.

Spoon the batter into the prepared pan and bake for 18 to 20 minutes until clean comes out the knife inserted in the center.

Cook the muffins in the pan for 5 minutes, then switch onto a cooling rack with wire.

Nutrition:

Calories: 125g

Fat: 115.g

Protein: 3.5g

Carbs: 3g

Fiber: 1.5g

Carbs: 11.5g

Chocolate Protein Pancakes

Preparation Time: 5 minutes

Cooking Time: 15 minutes

Servings: 6

Ingredients:

1 cup canned coconut milk

¼ cup coconut oil

8 large eggs

2 scoops (40g) egg white protein powder

¼ cup unsweetened cocoa powder

1 teaspoon vanilla extract

Liquid stevia extract, to taste.

Directions:

In a food processor, add the coconut milk, coconut oil, and eggs.

Pulse the mixture several times and then add the other ingredients.

Mix until smooth and well–change sweetness to taste.

Heat medium-heat a non-stick skillet

Using about 1¼ cup per pancake, spoon in batter

Cook until bubbles form at the batter's surface, then flip carefully.

Let the pancake cook until it browns on the underside.

The leftover batter is moved to a plate to keep warm and repeat.

Nutrition:

Calories: 455g

Fat: 38.5g

Protein 23g

Carbs: 8g

Fiber: 3g

Net carbs: 5g

Beef and Eggplant Kebab

Preparation Time: 20 minutes

Cooking Time: 15 minutes

Serving: 4

Ingredients:

- 3 tbsp. oil
- 1/2 tsp. dried thyme
- 1/2 tsp. oregano
- 2 eggs (beaten)
- 1/2 eggplant
- 1/2 tsp. chili pepper (ground)
- 1/4 cup olive oil
- 4 garlic cloves (crushed)
- 1 cup parsley leaves (chopped)
- 1 lb. beef (minced)
- 1 tsp. salt
- 1/2 tsp. black pepper

Directions:

1. Cut the eggplant into thin slices of about half inch. Season with salt and set aside. Put minced meat in a large bowl, add thyme, eggs, chili pepper, onions, parsley, olive oil, garlic, salt, oregano, and black pepper.

2. Combine the mixture. Shape equal-sized patties with wet hands. Preheat a skillet over medium-high heat and grease with oil. Rinse the eggplant slices sprinkled with salt and pat dry with hand or paper towel. Thread eggplant slices and patties alternately onto skewers and place on the preheated skillet.
3. Flip the sides occasionally and cook for 15 minutes. Remove from the heat and garnish with parsley. Serve warm with low-carb pita bread.

Nutrition:

39g Fat

23g Protein

4g Net Carbs

465 Calories

Skin Salmon with Pesto Cauliflower Rice

Preparation Time: 20 minutes

Cooking Time: 20 minutes

Serving: 3

Ingredients:

- 3 cups frozen riced cauliflower
- 1/cup olive oil
- 1 lemon
- 1 scoop Ketogenic MCT powder
- 1/4 cup hemp hearts
- 3 garlic cloves
- 3 salmon fillets
- 1 tbsp. butter
- 1 tbsp. olive oil
- 1 tbsp. coconut amino
- 1 tsp. red boat fish sauce
- 1 cup basil leaves (chopped)
- 1/2 tsp. pink salt
- Pinch of salt

Directions:

1. Grease a dish with olive oil, add coconut amino and fish sauce. Pat dry the salmon fillets and place them on marinade with meat side down. Season the top with salt and set aside for about

20 minutes. Add the minced garlic, hemp hearts, lemon juice, basil, olive oil, MCT powder, and salt in a food processor.

2. Blend until it reaches a sauce-like consistency. Add olive oil to a large skillet and put it on the stove-top. Add the cauliflower rice and cook until crisp-tender. Scoop out a few spoons of pesto you prepared and add into the skillet. Season with pink salt and stir until fully incorporated.

3. Place a skillet on medium heat and line with butter. Add the salmon with skin side down and cook for 5 minutes or until the crust browns. Flip the side and coat it with the remaining marinade. Sauté for about 2 minutes and remove from heat. Dish out the salmon and cauliflower rice. Top with pesto and serve warm.

Nutrition:

51 g Fat

33.8g Protein

10g Net Carbs

647 Calories

Chicken Enchilada Casserole

Preparation Time: 5 minutes

Cooking Time: 40 minutes

Serving: 6

Ingredients:

- 1/4 tsp. xanthan gum
- 1/2 tsp. onion powder
- 1 tsp. chili powder
- 1 tsp. cumin
- 1 tsp. garlic powder
- 1 tsp. oregano
- 6 lbs. chicken breast (boneless)
- 2 oz. black olives (slivered)
- 2 cups chicken broth
- 4 oz. green chilies
- 3/4 cup sour cream
- 1 cup cheddar cheese
- 3 tbsp. butter
- 1/2 tsp. pink Himalayan salt

Directions:

1. Place a large skillet over medium-high heat and add butter. Add the xanthan gum and allow thickening. Pour the chicken broth and stir through the xanthan gum. Allow cooking for

two minutes. Sprinkle with salt, onion powder, olive, cumin, and oregano, and chilies. Stir thoroughly to combine.

2. Add the chicken and bring to boil. Low the flame and allow cooking for 20 minutes with the lid on. Stir occasionally to avoid sticking. Remove from heat once the chicken is fully cooked. Shred the cooked chicken into small chunks. Place a skillet over medium heat and add in the sour cream. Stir in the spices to taste and add the shredded chicken. Preheat the oven to 350°F. Season with cheddar cheese and transfer the skillet to the oven. Bake for 10 minutes or until the cheese melts. Serve warm with cauliflower rice or tortillas. Keep in an airtight container to refrigerate for up to two weeks.

Nutrition:

20.7g Fat

27.8g Protein

4.5g Net Carbs

309 Calories

Ketogenic Cottage Pie

Preparation Time: 15 minutes

Cooking Time: 45 minutes

Serving: 10

Ingredients:

Base

- 2 pounds beef (minced)
- 3 celery sticks (chopped)
- 1 onion (chopped)
- 1 tbsp. dried oregano
- 2 garlic cloves (ground)
- 3 tbsp. olive oil
- 3 tbsp. tomato paste
- 1 cup beef stock
- 1/4 cup red wine vinegar
- 2 tbsp. dried thyme leaves
- 10 ounces green beans
- 1 tsp. salt

Topping

- 3 ounces butter
- 1 pinch of dried oregano
- 3 eggs (only yolk)
- 1/4 tsp. pepper (ground)
- 6 pounds florets of cauliflower

- 1 pinch of paprika
- 1/2 tsp. salt

Directions:

1. Put a large skillet over medium-high flame. Add olive oil, oregano, onion, celery, and garlic. Grill for 5 minutes or until the onion becomes translucent. Add the minced beef and sprinkle salt. Stir occasionally till the meat begins to brown. Add tomato paste to the cooked meat and mix well. Pour the beef stock and red wine vinegar.
2. Allow stewing for 20 minutes till the stock and vinegar evaporate. Add thyme and green beans and cook for another 5 minutes. Use a slotted spoon to dish out the mixture and set aside.
3. Take a large saucepan and fill two-third of it with water. Cover the pan and heat till the water begins to boil. Add the cauliflower florets to boiling water. Simmer for about 7 minutes until it tenders. Discard the cooking water carefully.
4. Add butter, pepper, and salt to the saucepan containing drained cauliflower. Mash the

tendered cauliflower by stick blender. Add egg yolks to the mashed cauliflower and mix well.

5. Preheat the oven to 350°F. Grease the baking dish with butter and transfer the minced beef mixture to it. Top it with cauliflower mash. Garnish with oregano and paprika. Bake in preheated oven for half an hour or until the top starts to brown. Serve immediately or refrigerate for up to 7 days.

Nutrition:

36g Fat

18g Protein

4g Net Carbs

420 Calories

Pan Fried Spinach Stuffed Chicken

Preparation Time: 10 minutes

Cooking Time: 20 minutes

Serving: 2

Ingredients:

- 1 tbsp. mozzarella cheese (grated)
- 2 tbsp. cream cheese
- 1 chicken breast (boneless)
- 1 tbsp. onion (chopped)
- Oil as needed
- 1 tbsp. butter
- 1/2 cup spinach (chopped)
- Salt to taste
- Pepper to taste

Directions:

1. Place a pan over medium-high heat and add butter. Add onions and spinach, allow to cook for two minutes or until cooked thoroughly. Add in the cream cheese to the pan, mix well to combine. Allow simmering for two minutes.
2. Lay the chicken flat on your cutting board. Use a sharp knife to deep cut a pocket through chicken breast. Flavor both sides of chicken

with salt and pepper. Spoon the shredded cheese and spinach mixture into the pocket.
3. Fold and seal the chicken breast with toothpicks. Place a skillet over medium-high heat and add olive oil. Cover the pan with a lid and cook the chicken for 8 minutes or until golden. Cut through the middle and serve hot.

Nutrition:

15g Fat

27g Protein

255Calories

Ketogenic Chicken Tenders

Preparation Time: 10 minutes

Cooking Time: 30 minutes

Serving: 6

Ingredients:

- 1 egg
- 1 lb. chicken breast tenders
- 1 tbsp. heavy whipping cream
- 6 oz. buffalo sauce
- 1 cup almond flour
- Salt to taste
- Pepper to taste

Directions:

1. Preheat the oven to 350°F. Marinate the chicken tenders with salt and pepper. Crack the egg into a small bowl and beat it with heavy cream. Mix the almond flour with salt and pepper in a zip-top bag or mixing bowl.
2. Dip the marinated tender in the egg and then in the almond flour. Repeat the process with all tenders. You can also coat the tenders by shaking them in a Ziploc bag filled with almond flour. Ensure the tenders are well coated with almond flour.

3. Use the fork to place tenders on a baking sheet greased with oil. Place the sheet in the oven and allow to bake for 30 minutes or until the crust browns. Remove from the oven and allow to cool. Add buffalo sauce and tenders in a Tupperware container and shake gently for proper coating. Transfer to the serving plate and enjoy the delicious chicken tenders.

Nutrition:

14.7g Fat

29.3g Protein

285 Calories

Low-Carb Salmon Tray Bake

Preparation Time: 5 minutes

Cooking Time: 15 minutes

Serving: 2

Ingredients:

- 2 medium salmon fillets
- 1 bunch broccolini
- 1 tbsp. extra virgin olive oil
- 2 tsp. whole-grain mustard
- 4 tbsp. Paleo mayonnaise
- 2 tsp. Dijon mustard
- Salt, to taste
- Black pepper, to taste
- Lemon wedges, to serve

Directions:

1. Preheat the oven to 200°C. Lay the broccolini on a cutting board and trim off the inedible parts — place in a baking tray and drizzle with olive oil. Pat the salmon fillets, and sprinkle the top with Dijon and whole-grain mustard.
2. Lay the salmon and lemon wedges with broccolini in the tray — season with salt and pepper. Bake for about 10 minutes until salmon is evenly-cooked, and broccolini turns tender-

crisp. Serve instantly with mayonnaise or store in the refrigerator for one day.

Nutrition:

42.5g Fat

34.3g Protein

552 Calories

Zesty Low-Carb Chicken Tacos

Preparation Time: 15 minutes

Cooking Time: 35 minutes

Serving: 4

Ingredients:

Tortillas

- 3/4 cup egg whites
- 1/3 cup water
- 1/3 cup water
- 1/4 cup coconut flour
- 1/4 cup almond flour
- 2 tbsp. avocado oil
- 1/2 tsp. salt

Filling

- 1 lime
- 2 cups lettuce
- 1 avocado
- 1 lb. chicken breast

Directions:

1. Preheat the oven to 400°F and line a baking dish with parchment paper. Place the chicken on a baking dish and bake for 30 minutes or until fork-tender. Add water, coconut flour, egg

whites, almond flour, salt and oil in a mixing bowl. Whisk together to combine.

2. Leave the batter to rest for 10 minutes till all the ingredients absorb well. Place a skillet over medium-high heat and grease with avocado oil. Take 1/4 cup of batter and add to the skillet. Spread the mixture with a wooden spoon.

3. Cook each side for about 4 minutes, flipping the sides occasionally. Remove from the heat once cooked thoroughly. Prepare all four tortillas by the same process. Place each tortilla on a separate parchment sheet and allow cooling. Slice the lettuce, avocado, and lime. Add the lettuce and avocado to the chicken and season with lime. Stuff the tortillas with chicken and lettuce filling.

Nutrition:

22g Fat

30g Protein

348 Calories

Ketogenic Chicken Doner Kebabs

Preparation Time: 20 minutes

Cooking Time: 50 minutes

Serving: 4

Ingredients:
- 4 low carb tortillas
- 1-pound chicken thighs
- 1 tsp. paprika powder
- 1 tsp. cumin powder
- 1 tsp. ground coriander
- 1 tbsp. olive oil
- 1 tbsp. lemon juice
- 2 garlic cloves (minced)
- 2 tbsp. hot sauce
- 4 shreds of cheddar cheese
- 4 tbsp. Ketogenic garlic sauce
- 1 cup shredded lettuce
- 2 serves Ketogenic Lebanese salad (tabbouleh)
- 1/2 tsp. ground pepper
- 1/2 tsp. onion powder
- 1 tsp. salt

Directions:
1. Take a large bowl and add chicken, lemon juice, garlic, oil, and all the spices. Marinate the

chicken by keeping it in the fridge for 3 hours. Refrigerate overnight for better results. Preheat the oven to 390°F.
2. Brush the metal skewers with oil and assemble the marinated chicken on them. Place the prepared skewers on the grill rack lined with foil. Make sure the chicken is not touching the bottom. Flip the skewers periodically and bake for an hour or 50 minutes. Make sure the meat is cooked through.
3. Put the chicken aside and prepare kebabs. Take a tortilla wrap and fill it with tabbouleh, cheddar cheese, garlic sauce, and lettuce. Fill all four wraps equally with the same ingredients. Sliver the chicken and add to the wraps. Embellish with hot sauce and gently roll the wraps.

Nutrition:

38g Fat

33g Protein

538 Calories

Low-Carb Instant Pot Frittata

Preparation Time: 10 minutes

Cooking Time: 30 minutes

Serving: 8

Ingredients:

Frittata

- 8 eggs
- 1/2 cup spinach (chopped)
- 1/4 cup red onion (chopped)
- 1/4 cup bell pepper (diced)
- 1/3 cup heavy whipping cream
- 1/2 cup cheddar cheese (shredded)
- Pinch of black pepper
- 1 tsp. chili powder
- 1 tsp. sea salt

Topping

- 1/4 cup red onion (chopped)
- 1 avocado
- 1 tomato (diced)
- 2 tbsp. spring onion (slivered)
- 1 pickled jalapeno pepper (crushed)
- 1/2 cup sour cream

Directions:

1. Take a large bowl and beat together the eggs and heavy cream. Add the black pepper, chili powder, salt, spinach, onion, bell pepper, and cheddar cheese. Give a good mix until all the ingredients blend. Grease a 7-inch baking dish with olive oil and transfer the mixture into it.
2. Fill the bottom of the instant pot with 1 cup of water. Place a trivet over the pot to keep the baking dish above water. Secure the lid, and use the manual button to cook for 12 minutes on high pressure.
3. Leave for 15 minutes till the pressure releases naturally. Remove the lid, once the floating valve drops. Add in the chopped tomatoes, salt and red onion. Mix well. Top the frittata with avocado, sour cream, jalapenos, and spring onion. Slice and serve warm. Refrigerate the leftovers in an airtight container for up to 5 days.

Nutrition:

17.6g Fat

9.4g Protein

218 Calories

Balsamic Chicken Thighs

Preparation Time: 15 minutes

Cooking Time: 4 hours

Servings: 8

Ingredients:

- 1 teaspoon garlic powder
- 1 teaspoon dried basil
- 1/2 teaspoon salt
- 1/2 teaspoon pepper
- 2 teaspoons dehydrated onion
- 4 garlic cloves minced
- 1 tablespoon extra-virgin olive oil
- 1/2 cup balsamic vinegar divided
- 8 chicken thighs boneless, skinless
- sprinkle of fresh chopped parsley

Directions:

1. Combine the first five dry spices in a small bowl and spread over chicken on both sides. Set aside.
2. Pour olive oil and garlic on the bottom of the slow-cooker. Pour in 1/4 cup balsamic vinegar. Place chicken on top.
3. Sprinkle remaining balsamic vinegar over the chicken. Cover and cook on high for 3 hours if

you have a fairly new slow cooker. If you have an older slow cooker you may need to cook another hour. Sprinkle with fresh parsley on top to serve.

Nutrition:

285 calories

20g fat

2g fiber

18g protein

Chicken Marsala

Preparation Time: 15 minutes

Cooking Time: 5 hours and 20 minutes

Servings: 6

Ingredients:

- Cooking spray
- 1 1/2 lb. boneless skinless chicken breasts
- kosher salt
- Freshly ground black pepper
- 8 oz. Mushrooms, sliced
- 3 cloves garlic, minced
- 1 c. marsala wine (you can sub with low-sodium chicken broth in a pinch)
- 1/2 c. water
- 1/4 c. almond flour
- 2 tbsp. heavy cream, optional (to make the sauce creamier)
- 2 tbsp. chopped parsley
- Lemon wedges, for serving

Directions:

1. Spray inside of slow-cooker with cooking spray. Season chicken all over with salt and pepper and add to slow-cooker. Top with mushrooms and garlic then pour Marsala wine on top. Cover

and cook on low for 4 to 5 hours, until chicken is cooked through.
2. Remove cooked chicken breasts from slow-cooker. In a small bowl, whisk together water and almond flour and whisk into the sauce. Whisk in heavy cream, if using, then return chicken to slow-cooker. Cover and cook on high until the sauce have thickened, about 20 minutes more. Garnish with parsley and serve with lemon wedges.

Nutrition:

312 calories

5g fat

3g fiber

33 protein

Chicken Fajitas

Preparation Time: 10 minutes

Cooking Time: 3 hours

Servings: 6

Ingredients:

- 4 boneless, skinless chicken breasts
- 3 bell peppers, thinly sliced
- 1 onion, thinly sliced
- 1/2 (7-oz.) can diced tomatoes
- 2 tsp. cumin
- 1/2 tsp. red pepper flakes
- Kosher salt
- Freshly ground black pepper

Directions:

1. Place chicken, bell peppers, and onions in slow-cooker then pour over diced tomatoes. Season with cumin, red pepper flakes, salt, and pepper. Cook on low for 3 hours, or until chicken is cooked through.
2. Remove chicken from slow-cooker and slice into strips. Serve fajitas in tortillas with desired toppings.

Nutrition:

354 calories

13g fat
2.3g fiber
41.2g protein

Spring Beef Bourguignon

Preparation Time: 10 minutes

Cooking Time: 6 hours

Servings: 6

Ingredients:

- 4 lb. beef chuck roast, cut into chunks
- 3 tbsp. extra-virgin olive oil
- 1 c. red wine
- 1/2 c. beef broth
- 2 c. sliced baby bell mushrooms
- 2 large carrots, sliced into rounds
- 1 large onion, diced
- 2 cloves garlic, chopped
- 3 sprigs fresh thyme
- 3 sprigs fresh rosemary
- 1 tsp. salt
- ½ tsp. pepper
- 1 bunch asparagus, trimmed and quartered
- Chopped fresh parsley, for serving

Directions:

1. Heat a large skillet over medium-high heat. While it heats, toss beef with oil. Sear beef in batches, 3 minutes per side. Between each

batch, deglaze pan with some red wine, scraping up any bits with a wooden spoon.
2. Pour mixture into slow-cooker along with seared beef as it's done. To slow-cooker, add beef broth, mushrooms, carrots, onion, garlic, thyme, rosemary, salt, pepper and remaining red wine.
3. Cook on high 6 hours, until beef is tender. Thirty minutes before serving, remove herbs and add asparagus; cook until just tender. Garnish with parsley and serve.

Nutrition:

613 calories

39g fat

49g protein

Mexican Shredded Beef

Preparation Time: 10 minutes

Cooking Time: 9 hours

Servings: 10

Ingredients:

- 3 pounds beef chuck roast
- 1 onion, diced
- 4 garlic cloves, minced
- 2 tablespoons tomato paste
- Juice of one lime (1-2 tablespoons)
- 1 Tablespoon chili powder
- 1 teaspoon cumin
- 1 teaspoon paprika
- 1 teaspoon dried oregano
- 1 teaspoon kosher salt, plus more to taste
- 1/4 teaspoon red chili flakes

Directions:

1. Mix together the chili powder, cumin, paprika, salt, oregano and red chili flakes, set aside. Add the chopped onion and garlic to the slow cooker with the tomato paste, lime juice, and just 1-2 teaspoons of the spice mixture. Stir everything together until fully mixed.

2. Sprinkle the rest of the spices all over the chuck roast, patting to help it stick to the meat. Place the meat on top of the onion mixture and set cook on low for 7-8 hours. Total cooking time will vary for different roasts.
3. After meat has cooked, use two forks to shred the meat, removing any large pieces of fat or gristle as you find them. (If the meat is still too tough to shred, it needs to be cooked a little longer. Cook for an additional 30-60 minutes and check it again.) Stir to mix well with the sauce. Cover and continue to cook on low for another 30-60 minutes.
4. Before serving stir well again to mix the meat with the sauce. Taste meat and season with more salt to taste.

Nutrition:

416 calories

27g fat

28g protein

Pork Tenderloin

Preparation Time: 10 minutes

Cooking Time: 8 hours

Servings: 6

Ingredients:

Shredded pork:

- 3 lbs. Pork Tenderloin
- Salt/Pepper
- Olive Oil
- 1 Cup Chicken or Vegetable Stock
- 1/2 teaspoon Ground Sage

For blackberry sauce:

- 10 ounces Fresh Blackberries
- 1/4 Cup Balsamic Vinegar
- 1/4 Cup Olive Oil
- Pinch Salt

Directions:

1. Salt and pepper pork tenderloin. Sear pork in large pan over high heat. Oil the bottom of a 6qt slow cooker. Transfer pork tenderloin to slow cooker. Add stock and sage.
2. Cook on low for 8-9 hours. (I do not recommend cooking on high as it can cause the pork to dry out). Remove pork from slow cooker

and shred. It should be falling apart. Pulse blackberries in blender. Push blackberry mixture through mesh strainer. Discard seeds.
3. In a 3.5qt pot, bring blackberry pulp, vinegar, olive oil and salt to a boil. Reduce heat and simmer 15-20 minutes while whisking occasionally. Vigorously whisk the last 2-3 minutes.
4. Once the sauce reaches a syrupy consistency, set aside to cool and thicken for 10 minutes before serving.

Nutrition:

188 calories

11g fat

30g protein

Creamy Lemon Chicken

Preparation Time: 10 minutes

Cooking Time: 5 hours

Servings: 6

Ingredients:

- 5 chicken breasts boneless and skinless
- 6 tablespoons unsalted butter divided
- 1/2 teaspoon kosher salt
- 1/4 teaspoon coarse ground black pepper
- 1 teaspoon Italian seasoning
- 2 lemons juiced and zested
- 2 garlic cloves minced
- 1 cup half and half
- 1 tablespoon heavy cream.
- 1 tablespoon chicken base optional

Directions:

1. In a large cast iron skillet add 1 tablespoon of butter to melt on medium high heat. Add the kosher salt, black pepper and Italian seasoning to the chicken and add it to the pan.
2. Cook on each side for 4-6 minutes. Add the chicken to your slow cooker. Cover with lemon juice, lemon zest, garlic and the rest of the butter in pieces

3. Cook on low for 4 hours or on high for 2 hours. In a large measuring cup add the half and half, heavy cream and chicken base and whisk well. Add the liquid, mix, and cook an additional hour on high.

Nutrition:

465 calories

21g fat

50g protein

Asian Porkchops

Preparation Time: 10 minutes

Cooking Time: 6 hours

Servings: 5

Ingredients:

- 4 thick-cut boneless pork chops
- 1 small onion, chopped
- ½ c. low-sodium soy sauce
- 2 tbsp. Splenda
- ¼ tsp. ginger

Directions:

1. Add pork chops and onions to the crock pot. In a small bowl, mix soy sauce, Splenda and ginger. Pour over pork chops in the crock pot. Cook on low for 6 hours or high for 3-4 hours. May need to cook a little longer if your chops are frozen.

Nutrition:

306 calories

15g fat

24g protein

Sausage and Peppers

Preparation Time: 10 minutes

Cooking Time: 6 hours

Servings: 6

Ingredients:

- 5 to 6 medium cloves garlic finely chopped
- 2 large yellow onions halved and thinly sliced
- 4 green bell peppers halved from top to bottom, cleaned and thinly sliced
- 1 tablespoon kosher salt
- 1 teaspoon Italian Seasoning
- 1/4 teaspoon dried oregano
- 1/2 teaspoon crushed red pepper flakes
- 28 ounce can unsalted crushed tomatoes
- 1/4 cup cold water
- 1 bay leaf
- 1 3/4 to 2 pounds uncooked Italian Sausage Links Mild or Spicy
- chopped Italian parsley for serving optional

Directions:

1. Finely chop garlic. Remove the chopped garlic and onion to the slow cooker Slice bell peppers in half from top to bottom. Remove the ribs and any seeds.

2. Add the sliced bell peppers to the slow cooker along with the salt, Italian Seasoning, dried oregano, crushed red pepper flakes, 1/4 cup cold water and 1 can have crushed tomatoes. Toss until well coated and liquid is evenly distributed.
3. Remove about half of the peppers and onion mixture to a bowl. Bury the uncooked sausages in the middle and return the peppers and onions back to the slow cooker to cover the sausage. Add the bay leaf. Cover, set to low and cook for 6 hours.
4. The onions and peppers will give off a lot of water as they cook which will make the sauce liquid and spoon-able so don't stress that there isn't enough liquid. Top with some chopped parsley, serve hot and enjoy!

Nutrition:

381 calories

23g fat

33g protein

Low-Carb Beef Short Ribs

Preparation Time: 15 minutes

Cooking Time: 4 hours

Servings: 12

Ingredients:

- 4 lbs. boneless or bone in, beef short ribs cut crosswise into 2-inch pieces
- salt
- pepper
- 2 tbsp. olive oil
- 1 cup beef broth
- 1 cup onion chopped
- 3 cloves garlic minced
- 2 tbsp. Worcestershire sauce homemade
- 2 tbsp. tomato paste
- 1 cup red wine

Directions:

1. Heat the oil in a large skillet over medium high heat. Season one side of your short ribs generously with salt and pepper.
2. Place half of the ribs, seasoned side down onto the hot skillet and brown. Season the top of the ribs in the skillet with salt and pepper. Flip once

the bottom is browned. Remove and set aside while browning the rest of the meat.
3. Add beef broth to slow cooker and place short ribs into. To the same skillet add your remaining ingredients and bring to a boil. Cook for 5 minutes or until onion is tender. Pour this over the ribs in the slow-cooker. Cover and cook on high 4-6 hours or low 8-10 hours.

Nutrition:

604 calories

34g fat

6g fiber

5g carbs

65g protein

Zucchini Lasagna with Meat Sauce

Preparation Time: 10 minutes

Cooking Time: 6 hours

Servings: 6

Ingredients:

- 4 small zucchinis, ends cut off (you can sub two large zucchinis)
- 1 pound(500gr) cooked ground meat or chopped meatballs
- 1/2 cup of your favorite pasta sauce
- 8 oz. mozzarella cheese, freshly shredded (about 2 cups), divided
- 15oz (425gr) container of part-skim ricotta cheese
- 1/2 cup Parmesan cheese, freshly grated
- 2 eggs
- 1 tablespoon dried parsley flakes
- 1 teaspoon salt
- 1/2 teaspoon cracked black pepper

Directions:

1. Thinly slice (unpeeled) zucchini length-wise into thin strips, like lasagna noodles. It's easier to do this with a mandolin, but a large knife

works just fine. (It's OK if some are only a few inches long.)

2. Create cheese filling by combining 1 cup mozzarella cheese, ricotta cheese, Parmesan cheese, eggs, parsley flakes, salt, and pepper.
3. Create a layer of zucchini at the bottom of your slow cooker. (It's OK if pieces overlap.) Top zucchini with a rounded 1/2 cup of cheese filling, 1 cup meat, and 1-3 tablespoons sauce.
4. Continue layering zucchini, cheese, meat, and sauce until you only have enough zucchini left for top layer. (A 6-quart slow cooker will have 4-5 layers and a 4-quart slow cooker will have 6-8 layers.)
5. Before you add the top layer of zucchini, add whatever sauce, meat, and cheese you have left. Top with zucchini and remaining 1 cup of mozzarella cheese.
6. Cover, and cook on low for 6-8 hours. Turn off slow cooker and let rest for at least 30 minutes, so juices become more set.

Nutrition:

386 calories

23.4g fat

112g protein

Chinese Pulled Pork – Char Siu

Preparation Time: 10 minutes

Cooking Time: 7 hours

Servings: 6

Ingredients:

- 1 kg pork shoulder or loin
- 1 cup chicken broth homemade is best
- 4 tablespoons sugar free tomato sauce homemade is best
- 1 tablespoon tomato paste
- 2 tablespoons garlic paste
- 4 tablespoons soy sauce
- 5 drops liquid sweetener
- 2 teaspoons ginger paste
- 1 teaspoon smoked paprika

Directions:

1. Place the pork in the bottom of the slow cooker. Combine all remaining ingredients and pour over the pork, ensuring it gets underneath as well.
2. Cook on low for 7 hours. Shred the pork with a fork and stir through the sauce, cooking for a further 30 - 60 minutes until the sauce has thickened to your liking, or eat it straight away.

Nutrition:

392 calories

23g fat

31g protein

Garlic Butter Chicken with Cream Cheese Sauce

Preparation Time: 10 minutes

Cooking Time: 7 hours

Servings: 6

Ingredients:

For the garlic chicken:

- 2- 2.5 lbs. of chicken breasts
- 1 stick of butter
- 8 garlic cloves, sliced in half to release flavor
- 1 tsp. salt
- Optional (but recommended) – 1 sliced onion or 2 tsps. of onion powder

For the cream cheese sauce:

- 8 oz. of cream cheese
- 1 cup of chicken stock
- salt to taste

Directions:

1. for the garlic chicken:
2. Place the chicken (thawed) in the slow cooker. Add the butter to the slow cooker. Place the garlic in the slow cooker, dispersing it around so it's not all in one spot. Sprinkle with salt. Cook on low for 6 hours. Remove and place on serving platter

3. for the cream cheese sauce:
4. In a pan, put the cup of chicken stock (or liquid from the slow cooker). Add the cream cheese and salt. Cook over medium-low heat until the sauce is combined and creamy. Pour over chicken.

Nutrition:

664 calories

38g fat

63g protein

Spinach Artichoke Chicken

Preparation Time: 10 minutes

Cooking Time: 4 hours

Servings: 6

Ingredients:

- 16 oz. Cream Cheese softened
- 9 oz. Frozen Spinach cooked and drained well
- 14.5 oz. Artichoke Hearts chopped
- 1 tbsp. garlic
- 2 cups shredded mozzarella
- 3 lbs. boneless, skinless chicken (we used thighs)
- salt and pepper to taste

Directions:

1. Place the chicken in the bottom of a slow cooker. Salt and Pepper well. In a bowl, mix together cream cheese, spinach, artichokes, garlic and season with salt and pepper. Stir in mozzarella cheese. Cook on low for 4-5 hours.

Nutrition:

460 calories

10g fat

34g protein

Bacon Wrapped Pork Loin

Preparation Time: 10 minutes

Cooking Time: 7 hours

Servings: 4

Ingredients:

- 2 lb. pork loin roast
- 4 strips uncooked bacon
- 1 package dry onion soup mix
- 1/4 cup water

Directions:

1. Rub pork loin with the dry onion soup mix. Pour any leftover into the bottom of the crock pot (any that fell off on my cutting board I scraped into mine).
2. Wrap the bacon around the roast and place into the crock pot. Pour in the water. Cook on High for 5 hours or Low for 7.

Nutrition:

388 calories

19g fat

40g protein

Chicken Cordon Bleu with Cauliflower

Preparation Time: 10 minutes

Cooking Time: 45 minutes

Servings: 4

Ingredients:

- 4 boneless chicken breast halves (about 12 ounces)
- 4 slices deli ham
- 4 slices Swiss cheese
- 1 large egg, whisked well
- 2 ounces pork rinds
- ¼ cup almond flour
- ¼ cup grated parmesan cheese
- ½ teaspoon garlic powder
- Salt and pepper
- 2 cups cauliflower florets

Directions:

1. Preheat the oven to 350 ° F and add a foil on a baking sheet. Sandwich the breast half of the chicken between parchment parts and pound flat. Spread the bits out and cover with ham and cheese sliced over.
2. Roll the chicken over the fillings and then dip into the beaten egg. In a food processor, mix

the pork rinds, almond flour, parmesan, garlic powder, salt and pepper, and pulse into fine crumbs.
3. Roll the rolls of chicken in the mixture of pork rind then put them on the baking sheet. Throw the cauliflower into the baking sheet with the melted butter and fold. Bake for 45 minutes until the chicken is fully cooked.

Nutrition:

420 Calories

23g Fats

7g Protein

Sesame-Crusted Tuna with Green Beans

Preparation Time: 15 minutes

Cooking Time: 5 minutes

Servings: 4

Ingredients:

- ¼ cup white sesame seeds
- ¼ cup black sesame seeds
- 4 (6-ounce) Ahi tuna steaks
- Salt and pepper
- 1 tablespoon olive oil
- 1 tablespoon coconut oil
- 2 cups green beans

Directions:

1. In a shallow dish, mix the two kinds of sesame seeds. Season the tuna with pepper and salt. Dredge the tuna in a mixture of sesame seeds. Heat up to high heat the olive oil in a skillet, then add the tuna.
2. Cook for 1 to 2 minutes until it turns seared, then sear on the other side. Remove the tuna from the skillet, and let the tuna rest while using the coconut oil to heat the skillet. Fry the green beans in the oil for 5 minutes then use sliced tuna to eat.

Nutrition:

370 Calories

23g Fats

7g Protein

Rosemary Roasted Pork with Cauliflower

Preparation Time: 10 minutes

Cooking Time: 20 minutes

Servings: 4

Ingredients:

- 1 ½ pounds boneless pork tenderloin
- 1 tablespoon coconut oil
- 1 tablespoon fresh chopped rosemary
- Salt and pepper
- 1 tablespoon olive oil
- 2 cups cauliflower florets

Directions:

1. Rub the coconut oil into the pork, then season with the rosemary, salt, and pepper. Heat up the olive oil over medium to high heat in a large skillet.
2. Add the pork on each side and cook until browned for 2 to 3 minutes. Sprinkle the cauliflower over the pork in the skillet.
3. Reduce heat to low, then cover the skillet and cook until the pork is cooked through for 8 to 10 minutes. Slice the pork with cauliflower and eat.

Nutrition:

320 Calories
37g Fats
3g Protein:

Grilled Salmon and Zucchini with Mango Sauce

Preparation Time: 5 minutes

Cooking Time: 10 minutes

Servings: 4

Ingredients:

- 4 (6-ounce) boneless salmon fillets
- 1 tablespoon olive oil
- Salt and pepper
- 1 large zucchini, sliced in coins
- 2 tablespoons fresh lemon juice
- ½ cup chopped mango
- ¼ cup fresh chopped cilantro
- 1 teaspoon lemon zest
- ½ cup canned coconut milk

Directions:

1. Preheat a grill pan to heat, and sprinkle with cooking spray liberally. Brush with olive oil to the salmon and season with salt and pepper.
2. Apply lemon juice to the zucchini, and season with salt and pepper. Put the zucchini and salmon fillets on the grill pan.
3. Cook for 5 minutes then turn all over and cook for another 5 minutes. Combine the remaining ingredients in a blender and combine to create

a sauce. Serve the side-drizzled salmon filets with mango sauce and zucchini.

Nutrition:

350 Calories

23g Fats

7g Protein

6g Carbohydrates

www.ingramcontent.com/pod-product-compliance
Lightning Source LLC
Chambersburg PA
CBHW071111030426
42336CB00013BA/2042